300NDFitness.com

ISBN 978-1-365-66013-9

Author: Steven Wilmes
Editor: Michael Nease of NeaseMedia.com
Self-Published by Wilmes, LLC

Contents

DEDICATION

This booklet is for all those who have ever struggled to lose weight and couldn't. Mom and Dad, this program is especially for you.

PREFACE

After losing 62 lbs and 9 inches around my waist, I would see people at professional conferences, on the street or at parties and they would not recognize me. People kept asking me how I did it; how I lost the weight. One night at a party, someone asked me these same questions in front of my lady - Reiko. She said, "it's all in his new book." When we got home she told me I needed to write the book because so many people needed my help. A few weeks later we were at another gathering and someone asked me again "how did you do it?" and Reiko said, "you'll have to buy his book".

That night, I started writing this booklet.

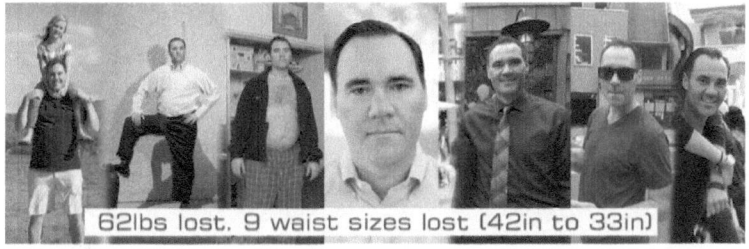

62lbs lost. 9 waist sizes lost (42in to 33in)

ACKNOWLEDGEMENTS

To Reiko: Thanks for all you encouragement and support during this journey, especially the big idea to write this booklet. You are truly my sunshine! And you really did save my life.

To Madison, my daughter: You are one of the best trainers in the world. Your level of mental toughness helped push me thru the hard parts of losing weight. At just 10 years old, you have the voice and strength of a veteran drill sergeant. Keep it up!

To Dr. Denise Herz: Thank you for giving me the heart rate monitor and the time to work on my fitness. You have given me a lot of support over the years. Thank you.

To my Mom and Dad: Whether you know it or not, all those comments about looking like Dad made me fear the worst.

To my little brother: I am still a hippie sometimes. Your sugar story was the funniest thing I ever heard, I wish we recorded it. Maybe you can.

1. MISSION

I'm on a mission and I want you to join me.

I want to help make Americans become more healthy and attractive.

As a whole, we as a nation are obese, or incredibly close to it. And to be honest, it's no fun to see obese people everywhere you go. Imagine what it would be like if everywhere you went, people looked good and healthy. I'm not talking about a world where everyone looks like elite athletes, but one where everyone ate within reasonable bounds and lived happy, healthy, active lives.

I want you to be healthy, fit and able to do the things you want to do. My mission for you is to help you achieve your fitness goals and be able to enjoy life to the fullest!

Here's the facts, this is more than just an issue of outward beauty, it's also an issue of resources. Bigger pants and shirts take more resources to make; bigger clothes weigh more and require bigger suitcases when you travel. This means we have to use more fuel to get the planes off the ground. On top of this, the extra weight we carry on our bodies leads to countless health issues ranging from diabetes to cancer. The resources required to care for these diseases, many of which are preventable, only makes the cost of healthcare increase, in turn bringing up the need and cost of health insurance.

Then comes the issue of waste. Bigger food portions require more resources to grow, process and transport. Sadly to say, most of this extra food gets thrown away in American restaurants. To what end? Here in California, we are experiencing phenomenal resource shortages and it's my belief that this is heavily due to our incredible habit of wastefulness.

As you will read in these pages, 300ND is not my attempt at creating some kind of new "fad-diet". In fact, it's not a diet at all but a return to a proper way of living. I believe with all my heart that this is a matter of life and death for all of us.

In addition, 300ND is my challenge for you to take the first step towards living the life you've always dreamed of living. It's my plan for you to be able to not only look great when you go to the beach in the Summertime, but to have the energy to play with your kids and live a long, happy and healthy life.

We're not creating something new here, just bringing something back that most of us seem to have lost somewhere along the way.

Are you ready to start making America beautiful again? Let me show you the way.

ARE YOU READY?

Are you ready to take back your life? Are you ready to see your feet again... Run like the wind... Jump over the tennis net on Saturdays and wear cool jeans again? What about walking into the room and having the other sex take notice of you or feeling light on your feet and walking without pain in your knees? Want to hang with the kids all day long? How about getting your cholesterol and triglycerides down, as well as lowering your blood pressure and increasing your chance of living a long life?

Sure we're doing this for us, but let's not kid ourselves... we like to impress others!

If you want to hear people say *"wow you look great"* or *"what the ... "*, *"I didn't recognize you"*, then you're definitely in the right place. By following the plan you're reading right now, I promise that I'm going to help you do it. In time, you'll hear those same words I heard from others and feel the pleasure of being fit again.

This isn't one of those books filled with theory. This is the story of how I lost 62 lbs and 9 inches off my waist without being a *weirdo freak* that no one wanted to be around. It's my real life plan which I started when I was 44 years old – Yes, you read correctly: 44 years old. This actually works and will work for anyone who puts it into action.

So, what's this program about? It's simple: 300ND is about losing weight.

That's it. Nothing more, nothing less. It's not about getting big and bulky, getting a ripped 6 pack or being some superhuman butt-kicker. It's about being healthy, fit, lean and ready to move. Once you learn how to be 300ND fit, you can start focusing on achieving feats of strength, challenging yourself with 20x goals and other cool things. Believe me, you'll want to do those things and more because you will feel so good about yourself that you'll want to show off for anyone willing to watch. And plenty of people will want to watch you. On top of this, sit-ups will become easier, you'll be able to touch your toes again and you'll be able to work on those fitness tests that were popular when we were in high school – vertical jumps, stretching, pull-ups, push-ups and much more!

At 45 years old, I am in the best shape of my life! And you will be too.

2. I WAS THE PROTOTYPICAL AVERAGE

AMERICAN MALE MESS

I grew up in St. Charles, Missouri just outside St. Louis, near a farming community and as a young boy, I was very active. At age 9, I would ride my BMX bike all around town, sometimes as far as 15 miles from my house to visit my aunt and uncle. I would organize baseball games among the neighborhood kids every day after school and we would play for hours. We had an in-ground swimming pool in our backyard and I swam every chance I got. Around 15, I would ride my bike to our family swimming pool business and work the shop. I would toss around 50lb carboys full of bleach and 100lb bags of sand for hours a day.

Then in a single bad decision, I picked up a cigarette and my healthy lifestyle was over. I was smoking a pack a day at 16 and by the time I was 20, I was up to 3 packs a day. When I turned 16, I got a used car and was able to grow a mustache. I quickly learned about beer and whiskey. And I also quickly learned that I could purchase alcohol for my buddies and make a few bucks while I was at it. Around the same time, the partying started and I was drinking with the best of them. Luckily, my metabolism was strong.

When I graduated high school, I weighed 145 lbs and looked sickly. I went to college, kept drinking and started eating all that nutritionless 'college food'. Without the physical job, the active sports or access to my swimming pool, within 2 months I had put on 40 lbs. I weighed 185 lbs on a 6'1 frame, but it wasn't 40 lbs of muscle, it was 40 lbs of beer belly.

Fast forward to my late 30's. I was a corporate junkie working late nights, driving every freeway known to man; sleeping in random hotels; spending two hours in California's infamous rush hour (the 405 and the 101) just to get home. Once I got home, I would settle in with six to eight Johnnie Walker Blacks on the rocks. Not to mention, I ate every snack that any of my co-workers put out at the office and couldn't wait to celebrate some random person's birthday because there was free cake and usually some high calorie lunch that I didn't have to pay for. I was a mess at just 39 years old. But don't get me wrong, I was this way at 35, 32, 30 and yes, even at 28. I idolized Tony Soprano from the hit HBO TV show and had the gut to prove it.

Heck, I even passed out three times from stress, and once because I was too dehydrated from drinking margaritas after spending the afternoon in Hermosa Beach trying to surf.

My wife (at the time) started to find me less and less attractive which didn't help my confidence at all. I sunk further – or should I say expanded further and further – into typical 'American bliss'. I was fat, unhappy and suffering from depression. I was taking it out on the wife, my beautiful daughter, the extended family, my boss, my co-workers and everyone around me. To put it bluntly: I was fat, unhappy and a complete asshole.

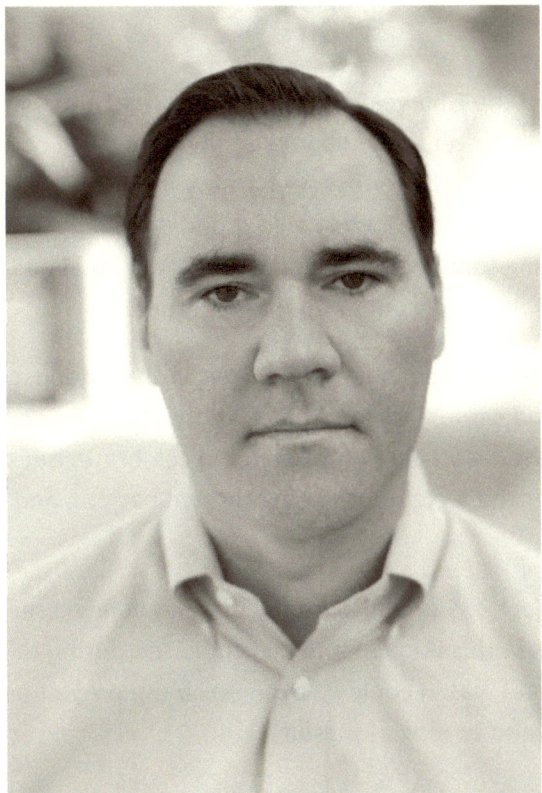

Me in 2012

MY TURNING POINT

I grew up in the Midwest were "big" is normal and bigger food portions the better. I would look at my father and could see his gut get larger and larger every year. My friends would say to me, "Wow, you really look like your dad!" Then my dad even began saying that I was starting to look like him. I had to do something, but just couldn't pull it together.

I tried the 'office version' of the Biggest Loser and lost 19 lbs in 6 weeks and came in second place at my office. My boss at the time bought me a new pair of pants to celebrate, but several weeks later the weight was being thrown back on and the pants didn't fit.

I tried project 365 (a photography project) you will see some of the photos in this booklet and all I could see during the project was how fat I was. I couldn't even finish the project because I couldn't stand to look at myself.

Finally, I tried the infamous P90X with some success but had to travel a lot for work. At that time, they didn't have portable videos available, so that fell apart on me too – my fault I know, but hey it didn't work for me either.

Then one day, at age 43, I had to take a 14 hour road trip to Arizona and I invited my dad to join me so we could spend some quality time together. At one moment during the trip, my dad and I were listening to Jim Rohn on a Success Magazine CD talking on the topic of health. Jim said that all you had to do to be in the top 3 percent of healthy people was to do the hard work. I looked over at my dad's belly which was easily 12 inches past my own and asked him – "Dad, do you think you are in the top 3 percent of healthy people?" to which he confidently replied, "Yes." Right then and there I knew I needed to do something or I was going to take on this 'Midwest mindset' and end up just as big as him.

I started looking for what I could do since I had tried nearly every program out there – Body for Life, Insanity, P90X and even the 10 minute workouts – and still, nothing had worked for me. I was falling deeper into depression and I hated myself but didn't have the motivation, the drive, or the skills to lose the weight but boy did I have excuses. More time slipped by – another 12 months to be exact before I finally found the breakthrough I was looking for.

Sound like you? Well today is 'No More Excuses Day'. Are you ready?

NO MORE EXCUSES

My 'No More Excuses Day' came in January 2015 when my neighbor Michelle bought a spin bike. I helped her put it together and that got me thinking again about my own health. At that time, I was already working on changing myself for the better. I wanted to stop cursing in front of my daughter, so I sought out hypnotherapy and that actually seemed to work. Then it hit me… I needed to get in shape.

I absolutely hated the thought of running and I certainly did not like the idea of spinning. But since Michelle was going to do it, I thought maybe I should check it out. A short time later, I stopped by a place called California Fitness and met a former NFL player who got me pumped about the idea of using a spin bike. They put me on a CMXPro by Cascade and I started pedaling. The seat felt great, the action was smooth and overall, I felt good about it. I couldn't believe it. Then I looked at the calorie count for the little bit of time that I was on the machine. *Unbelieveable!*, I thought. *I'm burning 50 calories in 3 minutes!* They assured me the readout was correct, but I couldn't wrap my mind around it. Right then, a voice of an elderly gentleman in my neighborhood started ringing in my head – "all I try to do is burn 300 to 400 calories a day." That was when it hit me – on this thing, I could do that in no time flat. It seemed too good to be true, so I had to ask again, "Is the calorie count on this thing correct?", "Oh, yes" they assured me. Then I looked at the price tag and split for the door.

A few weeks later on February 12th, 2015, I walked back into the store and climbed back on the CMXPro bike. This time they confirmed my previous suspicions and told me the calorie counter was off, but the bike still performed well and I liked the comfort. They cut me a hell of a deal on a new CMXPro bike and out the door I went. The rest is history, as they say.

At the time I'm writing this, it's been more than a year since I helped my neighbor put her bike together. I dropped the weight and she has not. The difference lies in doing the work just like Jim Rohn said in that Success Magazine talk. In his book "The Boron Letters", Gary C. Halbert explains through a series of letters to his son, "Everyone wants to climb the mountain, but the big difference between those at the top and those still on the bottom is simply a matter of showing up tomorrow to give it just one more shot." Don't be the one at the bottom. I know you're not, because you picked up this book.

All you have to do is start moving and keep moving, the rest will take care of itself. Part of it comes from how you set up your goals, so we will cover goal setting later in the book. Know this – you must take action. You must execute. You must do. And I am going to show you how. As we go through this book, I am going to share special quotes with you because it is part of the inspiration that I found helpful during my journey. In addition to this, you will need to find your own inspiration because you likely have different interests than I have. It's important that you make it a habit of continually seeking out that inspiration.

I am also going to get real with you and call out the things that will make you fail. I want you to succeed and I want you to look good and feel great. We have to get back to a place where Americans are more healthy and attractive, and that starts right here - with you and with me.

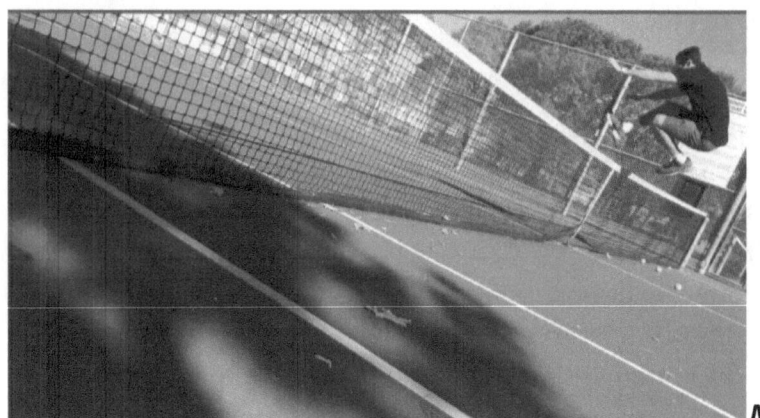

e jumping over tennis net – 36 inches

3. YOUR STRONGEST INFLUENCES

YOUR CIRCLE OF 5

"Anyone can put poison in your coffee, friend or enemy it doesn't matter... Watch your coffee". ~ Jim Rohn

We have to stop for a minute and talk about the people you spend the most time with. Countless entrepreneurs, authors, sales experts and motivational speakers all say the same thing: you are the average of the 5 people you spend the most time with. If those people are not supportive of your efforts to improve yourself, you may need to consider taking some time away from them. In some extreme situations, you may even need to consider getting new friends. Seriously, take a moment to survey your five closest friends and ask yourself if they're helping you improve yourself as a person. If the answer is "No", then it may be time to start surrounding yourself with new people who will encourage you as you move forward on your 300ND journey.

Whether you want to believe it or not, your friends may be dragging you down with them. Just like my mother and father keep each other in the "overweight / no exercise" circle, your friends will also influence you to either be healthy and fit or enjoy all the pleasures of life without control. Be very careful here. Willpower is limited and you don't want to use all of yours fighting this battle.

Your so called *friends* will pull you off track if they don't believe in where you want to go. Take some time right now, before reading any further, to fill out the list on the following page. Once you've done that, take some time to think about whether or not each person is a positive or negative influence on you.

It's important to identify the people who might pull you off track and what you should say to them when they try. This can even be as innocent seeming as your significant other telling you on weekend mornings to "Just sleep in a little longer". If *you* want this plan to succeed, you will need to continually remind these people not only of your goals, but that you need their support as you move forward on this journey.

MY CIRCLE OF 5

1. _____

2. _____

3. _____

4. _____

5. _____

NOTES

_____

_____

_____

_____

_____

ENVIRONMENT

Now that you've gone through your 5 closest friends, it's time to take a good hard look at your environment. Keeping junk food in the house, eating out several nights a week, taking your kids to fast food restaurants or eating the cake in the breakroom all have the ability to quickly pull you off track. You may need to change things up, especially if you aren't a person with great willpower.

In his book, *The Miracle Morning,* Hal Elrod points out, "If you don't have the willpower to turn off the alarm in the morning, it's simple, just move the alarm clock across the room." If you really want these changes to last, you're going to need to make some significant changes to your environment and find a way to hold yourself accountable (even it if means hiring me to call you every day). The best part about this (I've personally experienced it) is that you can bounce back from *years* of bad decisions. I did it and you're about to as well. The body is an amazing piece of machinery and 300ND is your answer to getting yourself back on track so you can start tuning it up again.

If you follow this plan consistently, I can guarantee that you're going to see results; the key is keeping the results after your get them. If you don't want to revert back to the way things were, there are two core factors that you need to be aware of – environment and accountability. We just covered environment, now let's dig in to accountability.

ACCOUNTABILITY

"Be Obsessed or Be Average" ~ Grant Cardone

Accountability to yourself, for yourself and by yourself is going to be the main objective for your long term success. We often cannot rely on the people immediately around us to hold us to a standard that they really don't care about and that you don't really care about. Once you make it hard for them to hold you accountable, most will give up on you, and when that happens, guess who goes back to ground zero?

You do.

You may be thinking, *I've tried that and it doesn't work*. Believe me, you are not alone in this.

This then begs the question, *Where can I find a reliable source of accountability?* In almost every circumstance, your best option is going to be finding a public option that you pay for. If you're the type of person who can't hold themself accountable, then you're going to need to put your money where your mouth is and invest in a proven accountability program.

Our 300ND accountability program is designed around this concept and while there are easily dozens of other groups out there, ours is specifically crafted around the 300ND philosophy and way of life. Regardless of which program you choose, make sure you find one with accountability as one of its key focuses and an active community of people who are excited to knock you around if you don't hold up your end of the bargain.

Here are some additional ideas for accountability. It's important that you make these difficult so you don't just give up on them:

- Ask your boss to not give you a raise if you don't meet your goals.
- Ask your wife or husband or significant other to withhold sex or stop doing your favorite thing for you.
- Let your significant other order your food when you go out if you don't meet your activity goals.
- Bet someone (hopefully someone that loves to see you lose) some cash.
- Tell all your coworkers what you are up to.
- Commit to a charity.

It's time to get real! This is a life or death matter – staying obese will kill you!

Don't be average, don't be the one at the bottom of the mountain. Get serious, change your environment and find someone to hold you accountable in addition to yourself. You can find out more about our 300ND Accountability Program on our website 300NDFitness.com.

4. THERE IS NO OVERNIGHT SUCCESS

"No one can see in the work of the artist how it has become." ~ Nietzsche

When I began my weightloss journey, I was a long way off course and it took me a long time to find my way back to a healthy lifestyle. I didn't magically drop 62lbs, although, looking back it sure feels that way. The reality is, it was a long, slow burn that got me to the point where I was ready to take action. It was the dedication to working out, eating right and the ups and downs involved with all of it that got me here. Get your mind right – it's going to take time.

Most likely you are just like me in that respect, you need time to think things over, try different options and then when you start to see results, you get excited and dive head first into it. I didn't know it at the time, but that is exactly what 300ND is – the perfect remedy to the long road ahead. The ultimate answer. The last word in weight loss fitness.

"With everything perfect, we do not ask how it came to be. We rejoice in the present fact as though it came out of the ground by magic."
Nietzsche

To help you find the same success I have found, I want to share the secrets and keys of my weightloss journey with you. These are things that I read and did that made a lasting impact and contributed to my overall success. Due to the mess that I was in at the start, I had lost almost all of my personal confidence and had completely stopped trying new experiences. This in turn lead to even less confidence, more depression, more dislike of myself and seriously negative thoughts. At one point, it escalated to the point where I nearly became suicidal. With the support of people I've never met, reading their books, listening to their podcasts and taking on their challenges, I found the strength to become the best version of myself I could be – at least for now. As my therapist Lillian Devin once said "it's not a midlife crisis, it's a midlife development." Yes, I did therapy. She was 100% correct.

You are about to embark on a long journey with very high peaks and very low valleys. Knowing that it is exactly the road you must travel will help drive you to success. Remember this quote from the movie The International – sometimes you meet destiny on the road you took to avoid it. You picked up this book because you have met destiny and you don't like it. Now it's time for our midlife development. Let's look this in the eye together and beat it.

For me it started with a new year. I didn't make any particular resolutions, but told myself I wanted to be an all-around better person. I had been reading tons of blogs on happiness, grit and mental toughness. That's when it really hit me. I was cursing like a sailor and had lost the reason why I cursed in the first place. I was doing this in front of my 8 year-old daughter and I wasn't the father I wanted to be. I took the alternate route and sought out a hypnotherapist to help me stop cursing. After one session (I bought into the idea of it) I had reduced my cursing considerably. By the end of the first week I was done cursing and by the end of the second week I was noticing that my level of anger and depression was disappearing. It's amazing the amount of hatred and anger that is concealed inside the "F" bomb.

After curing my profanity problem, I moved on to dealing with negative thoughts. Thanks to Mark Devine's book *The Unbeatable Mind*, I learned the power of finding my why and also coming up with a power statement to use when my mind started working against me. Your mind will work against you too, so learning some of these techniques will help you build grit and stick to the program, especially when the going gets really tough. And it will. Acknowledging it early is what is going to carry you through it.

I layered on the techniques from the book *The Happiness Trap* and learned how to deal with negative thoughts instead of trying to control them. You can't control thoughts from entering into your head, but you certainly cannot give them any weight or power over you either. You will experience negative thoughts and you're going to need to know how to deal with them. Pick up those resources and start reading them while you are waiting for the kids at their classes, running on the treadmill, spin bike or other machine. Read, read, read.

After gaining some knowledge about how to best deal with negative thoughts, I moved onto determining what my poor and rich habits were as Thomas Corley described in his book *Rich Habits*. He was right that if you enter in one rich habit, you will knock out 3 or 4 poor habits. That was the magic; instead of watching TV, I exercised. This made me thirsty, so I started drinking more water and it made me tired, so I started getting the 7-8 hours of sleep I really needed. I was also full from drinking water and didn't want to ruin my progress, so I started watching the calories I was taking in and burning off. Since I was drinking water, I wasn't drinking as much soda. Without soda, I stopped craving candy bars, ice cream and all the other sugary stuff.

You may not see the success when you eat healthy today, but you have to believe that it is helping you achieve your ultimate goal. Don't deviate when you don't see the results right away. The results will come, just maybe not as fast as you'd like. ~ Ryan Michler

The takeaway point here is that you have to focus on the PROCESS and not the end goal. Your goal has to be: doing the activity, not reaching some target. Change your goal to a process, make the process the goal and the result will be getting into great shape.

Example: Your goal is to lose 35lbs, how do you measure that? You must lose weight every day, but depending on the time of day that you get on the scale and what you did the night before, your weight may go up or down a few pounds and that sets you up for failure.

The Alternative: Instead of focussing on the activity, if you work out 30 minutes per day or burn 300 calories each day, the weight loss will take care of itself. By doing this, you will always find that you have accomplished your goal for the day, week, month and year.

This is the power of focusing on the activity rather than the results of the activity, which vary day to day. Think of it as a stock chart – it goes up and down every day, but over the course of a month, the value inches up and up. In your case, your weight and waist will be inching down and down.

I know you're probably thinking that all of the best books on setting goals focus on achieving results and how activity is just busy work. That is true for business, marriage and the like. Regardless, you have to do the right things. For fitness and weight loss, you need to burn calories and that means increasing your activity.

Activity equals calorie loss which equals weight loss.

This isn't rocket science, but it's critical to your success.

Novelist John Irving said it best in that "to do anything really well, you have to overextend yourself," to appreciate that, "in doing something over and over again, something that was never natural becomes almost second nature,". Finally, it's important to understand that the capacity to do work at this level of diligence "doesn't come overnight."

"We are what we repeatedly do. Excellence, then, is not an act, but a habit. ~Aristotle"

5. EQUIPMENT

NO EQUIPMENT

Many people think that they need fancy, expensive equipment in order to get in shape, but you don't have to look very far to realize that just isn't true. Just take a look at men and women in prison who manage to get in shape in spite of not having access to any of this overpriced equipment and you'll realize you don't need it either. All you need to do is just focus on doing the work.

I love equipment. My Ex-Wife used to call me an accessory king. For every idea that I had, hobby I got into or job task that I needed to complete, I would purchase every accessory known to man. Exercise was no different. When I joined a gym, I bought a new bag, new shoes, new shirts, shorts, sweat bands, water bottle and locks for the locker room. I even had a nice shower kit to go along with it all. When I got a new job, I bought the fancy pen, desk organizer and all kinds of other stuff I didn't really need. Then, I would spend so much time admiring all the stuff that I never got down to doing the work. Eventually, my closet was overflowing with junk and I would sell it for pennies on the dollar on eBay or just end up giving it away. What a waste.

Forget the equipment - it's nothing more than a distraction and a waste of money. With 300ND, you won't need any of it anyway. You don't need the fancy quick-dry shirts, the ultra-lightweight shoes, the fancy sunblock hat, or the designer socks. What you need is to simply get out and get moving, or as Nike says *"**Just Do It.**"*

EQUIPMENT (IF YOU REALLY MUST)

If you're one of those people like me who must absolutely get a piece of equipment to start 300ND, then let me recommend the single best thing you can buy for yourself. Go out and get yourself a proven activity tracker and heart rate monitor. There's a lot of options out there, but my personal favorite are the heart rate monitors and watches from Polar. If you can afford it, pick up the M400 or V800and if not, then grab yourself the A360.

The only reason that I recommend this equipment is because you can accurately determine the number of calories that you burned which is the core element of 300ND. If you can't afford these, there are a variety of activity tracking apps you can download onto your smartphone like the Polar Beat App. These apps aren't as accurate, but still help you track your activity and calories burned without the heart rate sensor, allowing you to have a better idea of how you are doing.

I received the Polar H7 heart rate monitor as a gift from my Ex-wife and later purchased the M400. It made a huge difference for me in terms of accuracy, which enabled me to shave a few minutes off my workout time the more I used it. But keep in mind, I was still dropping weight before I got any fancy equipment. I have since upgraded to the V800 which offers a few more tests and better tracking, but the equipment doesn't burn the calories for me, I still have to put in the work!

6. THE FIVE CORE CONCEPTS

1. **No Drugs**

2. **No Diet**

3. **No Days Off**

4. **Burn 300 Calories Every Day**

5. **Limit junk food to 300 calories per day**

LET'S GET STARTED!

If you are a self-starter then you can stop reading the book right here and just use those five core concepts to lead you. They are simple and self-understandable. However, reading the rest of this booklet will help to cement them in your mind.

CORE CONCEPT #1 - NO DRUGS

Let's face it, drugs are a crutch and they will break your wallet. Plus, once you stop taking them all your results tend to disappear. Prior to starting my 300ND journey, I tried Creatine, L-Carnitine, Amino Acids, Hydroxycut, Proteins and a few other legal drugs, all without ever really seeing any results. This is most likely because I wasn't eating right, sleeping right or exercising right. So this time around, I didn't use any of these supplements. I wanted to go about this in a clean and natural way that would help me to achieve real results that I could keep forever. I wanted to get my youthful body back, and I achieved it! With this plan, you will too - all without drugs.

The beauty of 300ND is that everything your body needs is in the foods you eat. You don't need to buy any of these fancy supplements or have to carry them around in your briefcase or purse. And you certainly won't have to worry about messing up your schedule because you forgot to bring them on your business trip. You don't have to worry about buying a special drink container, buying a special blender or finding extra space on the counter. All you have to do is eat what you are supposed to eat – a balanced variety. **Core Concept #2** - *No Diet* covers this in more detail.

Unless your doctor has prescribed you medication or supplements, I don't recommend that you add anything in the way of supplements or drugs. You just don't need them.

But don't you need energy? Okay, I hear you. A big portion of this comes back to your diet as well. Start eating a good variety of real food and you'll find that you have more energy. If you need to know what that really looks like, go to a real authentic

Japanese restaurant or look up recipes online (try Cookpad). The food is real, natural, and contains a balanced variety.

If you need a shot of energy, then head over to the Japanese market and pick up some Yunker or Lipovitan. Again, much better than American energy drinks loaded with sugar, plus they work. If you are getting the feeling that I am anti-American or have a dislike for American food, I don't. I love America, it's just that some of the options are not very healthy. So eat it in moderation and you will be fine.

CORE CONCEPT #2 - NO DIETS

I am serious when I say that the second ND in 300ND means NO DIETS. I know you are probably thinking that's bull, there has to be a diet in there somewhere – and to some extent, you're right – but not in the way you think.

When the word diet comes up, many people think that cutting down their caloric intake to a NORMAL level is somehow a diet. The fact is, it's simply what you're supposed to do – a normal way of eating. I cannot stress this point enough - eating at a normal caloric level is not a diet!

So, what is a diet?

Google defines a Diet as the following:

Restrict oneself to small amounts or special kinds of food in order to lose weight.

Herein lies the problem for most people living in America today. The amount of food that we typically consume on a daily basis is way out-of-whack! Many people are eating as many as 7,000 calories per day, which is far from normal. Dropping our caloric intake to normal levels is not the same as "restricting oneself to small amounts". Instead, it is restricting ourselves to completely normal amounts that are capable of sustaining your body and your life over a long period of time. On the flip side, it also doesn't mean eating more than normal amounts in order to 'bulk up'. We don't have anything against people who want to bulk up, it's simply not part of 300ND. This is one of the reasons that this program is so successful – you can have weight loss without losing muscle because you are still nourishing your body properly.

Another big issue with the word *Diet* is the restriction to 'special kinds of foods'. *Atkinson, Paleo, South Beach* and *The Zone* all have serious restrictions to help you lose weight. Unfortunately, as soon as people go off these *diets*, many report eventually regaining all the weight they lost. I was one of those people. The reason for this is that your body is not meant to operate on these narrow food options; it needs the proper nutrition that comes from a variety of sources. Fitness expert Tommy Baker talks about this, specifically pointing out that this is why programs like *The Biggest Loser* don't work. Don't believe us, just ask the people who participated in *The Biggest Loser*.

Then there is the other type of restriction that most Americans are currently on – the picky eater diet. My mother is in her 60's and all she eats or has eaten most of her life is beef, pork and chicken. No fish, no lamb – nothing else. I always ask her, don't you get tired of eating the same thing all the time?

Most people in America have gone down narrow roads and inadvertently put themselves on a diet by only eating beef or chicken and leaving out all the other items that make up the food pyramid. I'm not telling you that you have to stop your current way of eating or the diet you already have yourself on, but what I am saying is that you need to realize that you are already on a self-inflicted diet that doesn't work. So, if you want to lose weight, you need to get your mind wrapped around NORMAL. And that means accepting 300ND's Core Concept #2: No Diets.

Let's take a closer look at the term *diet*. Eating the number of calories that you should eat and the variety of foods to supply your body with the nutrients it needs is not a diet. You need to consume the number of calories for your age, weight, gender and activity level that is deemed normal and healthy. (You can find this information by logging into MY 300ND at 300NDFitness.com and following the provided steps.) *Active* and *Mayo Clinic* also have good calculators for this. Eating the right number of calories is not a diet, it's eating what you should be eating to maintain a healthy lifestyle. Adding or subtracting calories is a diet. Our goal is to help you live this 'No Diet' lifestyle by eating the normal amount each and every day.

Now that we have that covered, let's take a look at what I was doing before I developed 300ND. Each day, I would get up and skip breakfast. I would stop at starbucks and get a large coffee, then I would add cream and sugar. I would then roll into the office and eat two or three breakfast bars (270 calories/ea) that came from my makeshift vending machine which I had set up to supply snacks for the entire office. As a 'snack', I would then eat two or three (500-750 calories) candy bars before heading out to lunch at some fast food joint where I would eat a big burger with fries and a soda (2000-2500 calories). Afterward, I headed back to the office where I would top off my work day by drinking five to six Cokes (840 calories).

After work, I would head home and cook a big dinner which typically consisted of one or more of the following: pasta, pizza, steak and potatoes, etc. (2000+ calories). Later in the evening, I would drink 6 Johnny Walker Blacks on the rocks (420 calories), eat some chips and salsa, a row of Oreo cookies and some licorice (another 500+ calories).

My daily grand total rang in at approximately 7,280 calories!

No wonder I was 62 lbs overweight and had a 42 inch waist! I was on the Typical American Diet, and all I really needed to do was drop the extra calories to see a huge difference in my weight and waist. Adding exercise to it made it both healthier and more sustainable.

Does this sound like you? If your answer is yes, it's time to get real.

LET'S GET REAL

Take a moment and tally up the calories that you are eating. Are you up to 7k a day? Even 5k a day is two or three times the normal amount of what you need. If you're really serious about getting your health and weight under control, you're going to have to make some difficult decisions. It all starts with getting the junk out of the house.

Go ahead, do it now. Walk over to the pantry and throw it out – you don't need it!

CRUCIAL QUESTIONS

There are two questions we must answer before moving forward:

1. How many calories do you need to consume to maintain your healthy weight?
2. What is a health weight?

Here's the quickest, dirtiest and easiest formula for determining the number of calories you need to consume each day:

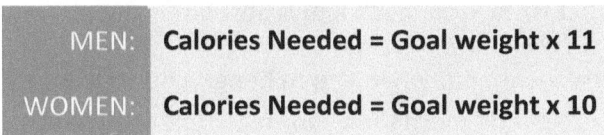

| MEN: | **Calories Needed = Goal weight x 11** |
| WOMEN: | **Calories Needed = Goal weight x 10** |

Example: For a man with a target weight of 183 lbs, your daily budget is 2013 calories.

To get a more accurate number, go to MY 300ND at 300NDFitness.com and look up the chart for the calories you need to be eating.

HOW MANY TIMES A DAY SHOULD I EAT?

This is a question that a lot of people ask me. Many so called 'Fitness Experts' will tell you that you need to eat 5 or 6 small meals a day. Your grandmother will tell you that you need to eat 3 square meals a day. Jillian Michaels in an interview with Darren Hardy for Success Magazine said you only need to eat 3 times a day, and two sentences later said that you needed to eat every 4 to 5 hours. At 4 hours, if I wake up at 5am and eat, then that's 9am, 1pm, 5pm and 9pm. That's more than 3 times a day. That is way too much and is absolutely not sustainable.

Here's the secret: eat when you're hungry, but make sure that you are not eating more than your recommended daily calorie count to maintain your desired weight. It's as simple as that. Remember, we have to keep this simple and sustainable. If you go to work every day or even travel for work, you cannot stop to eat every 2.5 hours (6 small meals recommended by those 'Fitness Experts') to eat a meal and you certainly cannot stay up 24 hours a day to eat once every 4 hours. We all have lives to live and while eating is important, it's not the only thing that we have to do. This is why other programs fail to help you achieve the results you are looking for, they simply aren't sustainable and are too rigid. That's the beauty of 300ND and why we can continue with this program for the rest of our lives.

CORE CONCEPT #3 - NO DAYS OFF

Sure Arnold Schwarzenegger is known for saying he had cheat days. I also understand that you don't want your body to think that you are starving it. But remember, we are not going on a diet here. We are eating what we are supposed to eat – the right amount of calories in the right variety. We are eating the foods we like to eat, in sufficient quantities to keep us nourished and healthy.

When you eat right, you don't need days off.

The beauty of 300ND is we are not tricking our body into thinking it is full. We are giving it the food that it needs to keep itself healthy and to give you the fuel you need to move, perform and maintain energy.

Okay, so you get that you don't have to take days off from a diet because there is no diet, and you realize that you don't have to take days off from supplements or drugs because 300ND doesn't use supplements or drugs. But what about the exercise?

The exercise portion of our program, which is a core component to getting you back in the best shape of your life, is simple to do and requires a minimal training load which means your recovery period is very short. Don't mistake simple, minimal and short for ineffective. This isn't a silly 1 minute workout, this is a serious sustainable program. You will sweat, you will be tired and you will feel the burn, just not in a way that beats you up so much you don't want to continue.

The next two core concepts cover two of the most crucial pieces of 300ND, but rest assured that you do not need to take a day off from the exercise program because it is a sustainable program that you can do anywhere, any time, every day. And your body will not only recover quickly, but it will thank you for it.

"To do anything really well, you have to overextend yourself, in doing something over and over again, something that was never natural becomes almost second nature." It "doesn't come overnight."

~ John Irving

CORE CONCEPT #4 - BURN 300

Julian Michaels, in a Success Magazine interview with Darren Hardy said "it's calories in and calories out" but that it is not easy to do. It's simple, but not easy. You have to burn the calories and you have to watch the amount of food you eat on a daily basis.

Why, if it is so simple, do so many people fail? The answer is easy to find if you look for it. It's always: *Time*. People simply complain that they don't have enough time. I know I sure didn't have the time. Even today my dental hygienist complained that she didn't want to go to the gym because she was too tired and didn't want to spend 1.5 hours trekking to and from the gym. Time is an excuse. You have to make time. Make it a priority and put it on your calendar.

That's why I needed something that was simple and sustainable. I needed something that I could do quickly and that I wouldn't get bored with. Something I could do at home, on the road, in Europe or Japan and at any time of the day.

The first 300 in 300ND is that you need to burn 300 calories every day. That's it, just 300 little calories every day. How you burn those 300 calories is up to you. You can swim it. You can walk it. You can run it. You can bike it. You can dance it, lift it, jump rope. Whatever you like to do, you need to do that. You can do it with your significant other/partner, your kids, your friends. I don't care just get it done.

We are not bulking up. We are losing fat. All we are going to work on is cardio – strength can come later and it will. Burn more than 300 calories today, that's cool – you are accelerating your weight loss.

How long does it take to burn 300 calories? That's a great question. It all depends on the activity that you are doing and the shape you are currently in. When I first started this life changing program, it took me four sessions of exercise to get to 300 calories. I was out of shape, tired and had no stamina. I got on the spin bike for 5 minutes and got off. Got back on and went for 10 minutes at a very slow pace. This went on until I burned 300 calories. The next day, I was dead tired, but I got on the bike and did what I could, then got off and came back to it later that day. This went on for the first two weeks. Then, magically, my body adapted and I was able to go for 20 to 30 minutes at a time.

By the fourth week, I was able to go an hour on the bike at a good pace without stopping. By the fifth week, I was able to burn the 300 calories in 30 minutes because I was able to go faster, burning more calories in less time. If you commit to this program, you will be able to do the same thing. You can burn 100 calories every 10 minutes jogging.

300ND EXERCISE EXAMPLES

Let's take a look at some activities and times for me to burn 300 calories. My VO2 max (the maximum rate of oxygen consumption as measured during incremental exercise) is 49, current weight 183, height 6'1" and Age 45.

Running – 27 minutes
Spinning – 25 minutes
Tennis – 30 minutes
Walking – 60 minutes
Krav Maga – 60 minutes

Here is a sample of times to burn 300 calories for a 155lb person published by the Harvard Medical School:

Activity	Time in Minutes
Frisbee	80
Volleyball	80
Horseback riding	69
Walking at 3.5 mph	60
Planting seedlings, shrubs	60
Planting trees	54
Badminton	54
Weeding	52
Hopscotch	49
Skateboarding	48
Playing with kids	48
Golf carrying your clubs	44
Cross Country hiking	40
Rollerblading	35
Tennis	35
Biking	30
Running	24
Jumping rope	24

MORE ON TIME

Time is the biggest excuse people give me as to why they haven't lost weight, and it's a total joke. Unfortunately, the joke is on them. Ever heard the phrase "make time"? What does that mean? There is no factory making time. It means that you have to make the things that are important a priority. In order for 300ND to be truly effective in your life, it needs to be one of your top priorities. Period.

Let's take a look at some of the ways you could take back some of your wasted time. Here are the top ways most people waste time every day:

- Standing in line at Starbucks instead of making coffee at home
- Watching TV
- Facebook, Twitter and other internet surfing
- Gossiping at work
- Going out for drinks
- Arguing with strangers about ideas that don't mean a thing to you
- Sitting on hold on the phone
- Driving around looking for the best parking space
- Watching the news
- Fixing things on the cheap and then fixing them again
- Buying too much junk and then having to organize it and re-organize it and then throw it away
- Hosting garage sales
- Serving on do-nothing committees
- Reading gossip magazines
- Running to the store multiple times a week, instead of making one big trip

Here's a bunch more from TimeManagementNinja.com

1. **Complaining.** No one gets what they want by whining. Instead, try asking.
2. **Commuting during rush hour.** Time-shift your drive for less traffic.
3. **Gossiping.** It never gets the work done.
4. **Doing other people's work.** Do your work first.
5. **Watching TV.** No one ever accomplished their goals by sitting on the couch.
6. **Hanging out with negative people.** Be careful, attitude is contagious.
7. **Procrastinating.** Action now always beats inaction.
8. **Indecision.** Make decisions or life will make them for you.
9. **Reading the news.** Go on a media diet.
10. **Antagonizing others.** If you don't have something nice to say…
11. **Playing video games.** Angry Birds doesn't get work done. Neither does Words with Friends.
12. **Eating junk food.** Do something active and get your body in motion.
13. **Making empty promises.** Stop saying what you're not going to do.
14. **Waiting for something to happen.** Go out and make it happen.
15. **Attending unnecessary meetings.** Practice the "Right to Decline" unneeded meetings.
16. **Reading Email.** Only check it 3 times a day. Morning, noon, end of day.
17. **Answering the phone.** Remember, *your* phone is there for *your* convenience.
18. **Playing Email Ping-Pong.** Avoid the back-and-forth, go talk to someone.
19. **Not putting things away.** You'll have to look for them later.

20. **Surfing the web endlessly.** One thing leads to another…
21. **Constantly updating your social media status.** No one needs to know what you are eating for lunch.
22. **Not capturing ideas.** Where did you write down that million dollar idea?
23. **Fighting with others.** Agree to disagree, but skip the fight.
24. **Reading the tabloids.** Do you need to know which celeb got arrested this week?
25. **Looking for things you misplaced.** Make sure you have a place for your stuff.
26. **Letting email notifications interrupt your day.** Turn off those pop-ups!
27. **Piling instead of filing.** Piles are not organization.
28. **Not looking at your todo list.** You wrote that task down, but you didn't look at your list.
29. **Solving the same problems, again.** Make sure you document solutions so you have them down the road.

And here's more evidence from Inc.om on time wasting junk:

About a year ago, the Harris Poll and CareerBuilder conducted a survey of thousands of managers and workers, hoping to find out the biggest time-wasters at work, and, in cases where people are choosing to slack off, exactly what they're doing to waste it. The results of the survey are both instructive and entertaining.

It's perhaps no surprise that the survey revealed that yes, people report a lot of wasted time at work. And the things they do or hold responsible are probably no big surprise either. Here are the top 10, along with the percentage of people who cited them as a cause of wasted time. As you can see from the numbers, many people listed more than one of these.

1. Cell phone/texting (50%)

2. Gossip (42%)

3. The internet (39%)

4. Social media (38%)

5. Snack or smoke breaks (27%)

6. Noisy co-workers (24%)

7. Meetings (23%)

8. Email (23%)

9. Co-workers dropping by (23%)

10. Co-workers putting calls on speakerphone (10%)

Even more interesting are some of the particularly novel ways that people have found to do anything they could at work besides *work*. Here are some of the best examples:

- Blowing bubbles in sub-zero weather to see if the bubbles would freeze and break
- Married employee looking at a dating website
- Caring for pet bird that employee smuggled into work
- Shaving legs in the women's restroom

- Lying under boxes to scare people
- Having a wrestling match
- Sleeping, but claimed he was praying
- Taking selfies in the bathroom
- Changing clothes in a cubicle
- Printing off a book from the internet
- Warming her bare feet under the bathroom hand dryer

The opinions expressed here by Inc.com columnists are their own, not those of Inc.com. Published on: Aug 20, 2015

If you are one of these people, you are also probably also one of the people who complain that you don't make enough money or didn't get the raise that you deserved. Well, your answer is listed above: stop wasting time! Let's face it, research shows that people with whiter teeth make more money, just like taller people and those that are in shape. Will 300ND help you make more money? It's possible, but only if you stop wasting your time. I told you that I was going to call you out. Be true to yourself and make 300ND a priority! You will thank yourself later.

SETTING GOALS

Setting goals for 300ND really does require that you understand how to set goals that matter. Most people subscribe to some form or another of Franklin Covey or SMART goal strategies. While this might be fine for your work life, it is not going to cut it for your fitness goals. The biggest reason is that you have to hold yourself accountable because no one else will. If you don't believe that, just ask yourself who has been holding you accountable and then look yourself in the mirror. That should be plenty of proof for you. Want more? If you were good at making and holding fitness goals, you wouldn't be reading this book, you would be writing it.

Your goals have to shift focus. You have to forget about results and zero in on activities. Losing 26 lbs is a great end result, but it is not sustainable by itself. You can't keep losing 26 lbs forever, and you certainly can't set that as a daily activity nor can you put a time requirement on it.

However, what you can put a time limit on is daily activity. You can exercise 30 minutes per day and you can burn 300 calories per day. The beauty of focusing on activities is that they stack up. As you do them, you will lose weight, build endurance and you'll feel great about yourself along the way. You can tick off your checklist each day that you burned the calories. That has to be your goal: Burning the calories.

GOAL: BURN 300 CALORIES

For the first 6 months of 300ND, forget about all other goals. You can add in dropping inches off the waist, smaller clothes, bigger arms, speed tests, jump height, endurance, power, weight lifting, trimming fat and all types of other things later on.

For right now – your goal is to burn 300 calories each and every day.

While I am really good at setting my own goals, I am not the best at convincing you to alter your mindset. I highly recommend that you follow in my footsteps and learn from the experts. People like Hal Elrod who wrote the Miracle Morning or Brian Moran in his book The 12 Week Year. These people will not only help you achieve success in fitness, but in all aspects of your life.

Just remember, focus on the tactics not the objective.

Your objective: loose weight.

The tactic: burn 300 calories every day.

BUSTING BARRIERS

Without a doubt you are going to face barriers when you start this program, especially if it's been awhile since you worked out. You may find that you cannot burn 300 calories in one session. You may have to bust your exercise into 3 or 4 sessions throughout the day. That's what I did, and I was proud to accomplish it. The good news is this usually only lasts for a week or week and a half. In his book *The Miracle Morning*, Hal Elrod explains that it is a formula of 10-10-10. This means that the first 10 days really stink, the second 10 are so-so and the last 10 you start to enjoy the new habit. Keep that in mind when you are doing 300ND. The first 10 days are tough and you will need mental toughness to get you through the second 10. After that you are on to a new life and a new better you.

There is probably no one better suited to teach you about mental toughness than Mark Divine. Mark, a former Navy Seal, gives this advice when trying to stick with finishing your workout program. Let's say you are running or jogging and you're tired and don't feel like you can make it any longer. Mark suggests that you start breaking down the exercise. No longer is it about burning 300 calories, now it is about buring 25 more calories. If 25 is too much, okay then break it down even further to just 10 more calories. When you get that under your belt, shoot for another 10 then another 10 until you finally break through and get your 300 calories.

Don't want to use calories as your metric? Break your 3 mile run into just another quarter mile. If that's too far, then get to the end of the block. Still too far? Just get to the end of the neighbor's yard, then past their driveway, then to the next house, etc... Read Mark's book Unbeatable Mind to learn more about this amazing mind and grit building technique.

CORE CONCEPT #5 – LIMIT JUNK TO 300

There is one more rule that is very important when it comes to 300ND and that is the amount of junk food you eat. You need to limit your junk food calories to 300 per day. Chips, candy bars, soda, cake, pie, Oreos, licorice, whatever it is, you can eat it, just don't eat more than 300 calories of it per day. Want to eat a little bit of a candy bar and some chips, go ahead, just limit it to 300 calories.

I know you are thinking – ah ha! See I told you there was a diet in here. Remember, junk food in excessive quantities is not a normal part of any healthy nutrition plan. In fact, added sugars are not part of the food pyramid.

Keeping your sugar or junk food intake at just 300 calories per day is part of Thomas Corley's Rich Habits which he writes about in his book *Rich Habits: The Daily Success Habits of Wealthy Individuals*. Thomas studied the wealthy and found that people who counted the calories that they ate and limited their junk food intake to 300 calories per day were able to maintain a healthy weight over their lifetime. The second part of this equation is adding 30 minutes of vigorous exercise; which is the First 300 in 300ND.

WHAT IS JUNK FOOD?

To get past the "that's not junk food" excuse, I want to clarify what I consider to be junk food. In order to keep with the 300ND plan, you will need to consider these things to be junk food as well.

Beer	Lattes
Whiskey	Soda
Potato Chips	Lemonades
Candy Bars	Ice Cream
Gummy Bears	Energy Drinks
Cake	Sugar
Pie	Trail Mix
Frappuccino	

Here is a great secret about junk food: If you really like this stuff and find that you just aren't getting your fill of junk food every day, then head over to a Japanese grocery store. Japanese junk food is not as sweet and has less sugar than typical American junk food. That means that the calorie count is much less, so you can get a little more volume out of your 300 calorie limit for the day. I am not encouraging you to eat more junk food, just letting you know that you have more options than you might realize.

HOW TO COUNT CALORIES

I am not sure how this happened, it could be a failure in the American educational system, but most of us don't understand how to count calories or what makes up our food. If you don't believe me, just look around and you'll learn that 60% or more of Americans are overweight and pushing obese. The evidence is there. I admit, I don't really understand all of the information listed in the labels on the back of food packages, but what I do know is that junk food is not a good source of calories. I also know that it doesn't matter the type of calories that you eat, they all count against you. So if you eat 900 calories of good quality food and 800 junk food calories, you still sucked down 1700 calories that you need to take care of.

So how do you account for them? First, forget about getting too specific. You don't necessarily need to get down to the smallest decimal, just focus in on the big stuff and round up those calories. This is especially helpful if you go out for lunch or dinner with someone; they don't want to sit around waiting while you're trying to figure out how many calories you just ate. It's important to keep it simple while remembering that 300ND is about not being a health-fanatic that no one wants to be around. It's simply about living a healthy, fit and enjoyable life.

There are a number of online and mobile tools that can aid you in counting and tracking your calories. One of the most popular is MyFitness Pal (available online and via mobile app), which has an extensive nutrition database from both store bought food and many popular restaurants. No tool is 100% accurate however, so don't obsess over it. These will get you close, and that's good enough.

UNDERSTANDING THE AMERICAN FOOD PYRAMID

Take a good look at the American food Pyramid graphic below. The purpose of charts like these is to try to simplify the information, but with how difficult it is to understand, they've clearly failed. It's no wonder that most Americans struggle with weight and weight loss. The Pyramid is so complex that it can't even be simplified into a single image and the yellow is not even labeled (it's oils by the way). At any rate, it is difficult to understand and I think most of us give up on it before we even get started.

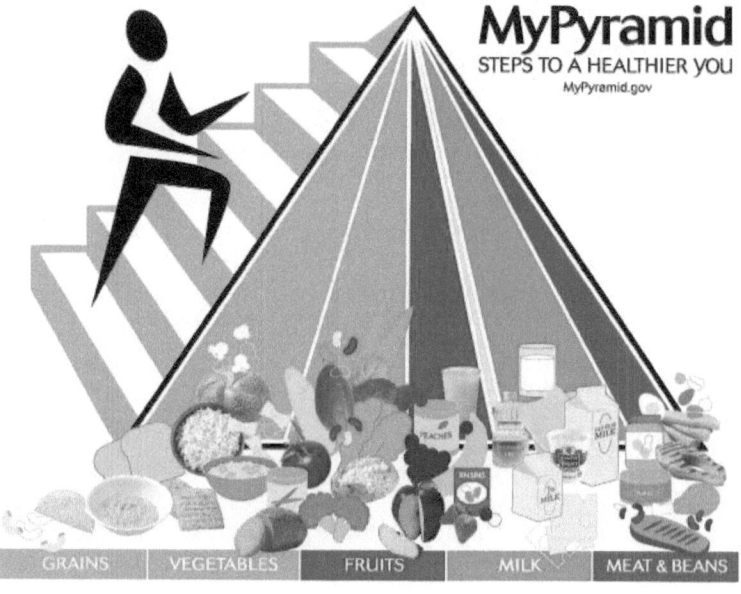

On the other hand, steps have been taken to simplify the image using ChooseMyPlate.gov. I like this version a lot better because it encourages people to eat real food, but , it still only provides one piece of the equation.

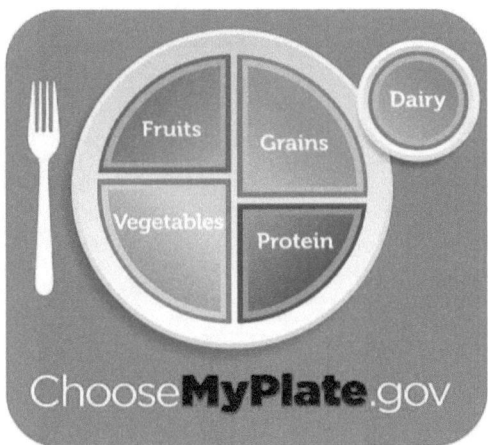

A HEALTHIER ALTERNATIVE

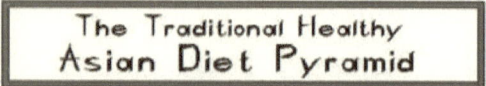

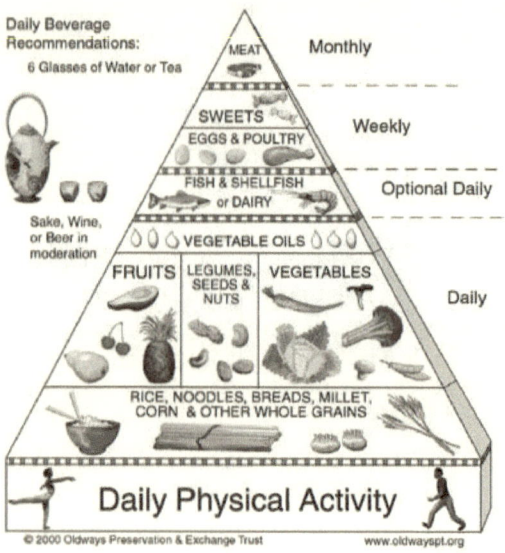

The Asian Diet Pyramid shows us a different structure of dietary priorities that exemplifies 300ND better than almost anything else I've seen. Maybe that's why if you travel to countries like Japan, you will find cultures of healthy, fit people.

Notice, that this pyramid doesn't tell you to cut out sugar entirely, but it also doesn't say to eat it every day. One of the most amazing parts (that is entirely missing from the other healthy living pictorials) is that exercise is built into the foundation this pyramid.

This Asian Diet Pyramid is very close to exactly what you need; however, if you want to have something a little bit closer to an American meal plan, then follow the Japanese and throw in a just a touch of meat here and there. Forget the big burgers and the steaks. Along this philosophy, meat should be used sparingly just like the other food groups in the pyramid. It should be a part of the meal, not the main course.

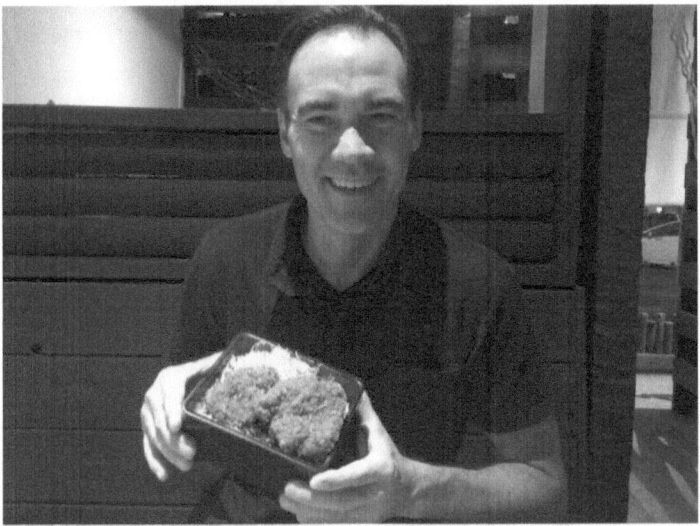

Fun Japanese food that tastes great

7. BRINGING IT ALL TOGETHER

300ND is a straightforward and sustainable program. No more, no less. With a program this easy, there's no reason you can't start changing your life today! It's time to get to it! Get out there and change your life for the better! Let's make this a nation of healthy and fit people once again!

You should now understand the 5 core concepts of 300ND: No drugs, No diet, No Days Off, Burn 300 and Limit junk to 300. Let's take a quick look at the concepts one more time. Drop the drugs (supplements): you don't need them, they are expensive and hard to manage. Forget the fad diets: Eat what you are supposed to eat in a good variety in real, natural foods. Figure it out by going to *My 300ND* at 300NDFitness.com. Forget about taking days off: You don't need days off because what we are doing is sustainable and easy on the body; We are burning fat and dropping weight. The two major keys – burn off 300 calories each day however you like in vigorous exercise. It doesn't matter if you have to break it up into multiple sessions, just get it done each day. Finally, limit your junk food to 300 calories max per day. Eat whatever you want in junk food, just limit it to 300 total calories per day. If you want to see better, faster results, then drop more of the fatty junk food.

That's it! Simple, easy and sustainable. Now the hard part is up to you.

Get to it!

You don't need any fancy tools, clothing or shoes; just what you have with you right now. No excuses.

Make sure you log back into 300NDFitness.com and follow the steps under My 300ND to figure out your daily calorie needs.

Write me and let me know how you are doing. Take a picture of yourself and post it at 300NDFitness.com We want to see how you are changing yourself to become more healthy and fit!

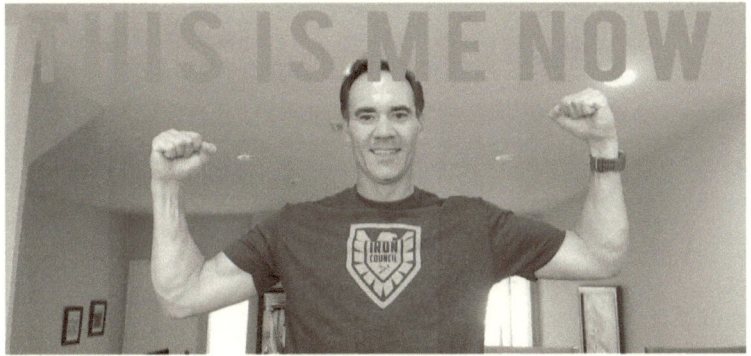

Don't forget to sign up for our Accountability Program

www.ingramcontent.com/pod-product-compliance
Lightning Source LLC
Chambersburg PA
CBHW020400290526
45785CB00005B/2373